Easy Separate Food Diet

A Simple and Effective Way to Lose Weight Without Hassle and Harm to Health

By Lydia Shkil

TABLE OF CONTENT

DEDICATION

This book is dedicated to every strong woman out there who like I was, is not in love with what the mirror tells her of herself.

I say to you that you are strong and I can see it; you are beautiful, inside and out. I can understand if you feel like I am ranting.

But this book is dedicated to you. Yes! To the 'new you' we will have, after you follow the instructions in this book.

It is dedicated to the surprise in people's eyes, and in the hope you'll give to other overweight women.

It is dedicated to the strength and tenacity with which you'll go through with this weight loss regiment.

And above all to the beautiful smile that will grace

your face.

purposes only. All effort has been executed to present accurate, up to date, and reliable, complete information. No warranties of any kind are declared or implied. Readers acknowledge that the author is not engaging in the rendering of legal, financial, medical, or professional advice. The content within this book has been derived from various sources. Please consult a licensed professional before attempting any techniques outlined in this book.

By reading this document, the reader agrees that under no circumstances is the author responsible for any losses, direct or indirect, which are incurred as a result of the use of information contained within this document, including, but not limited to, errors, omissions, or inaccuracies.

ABOUT THE BOOK

I confess to you that in this book- 'Easy Separate Food Diet', the method I will describe, is somewhat not your regular separate feeding theory. This is different from the principle of separate feeding founded by Herbert M. Shelton in 1928.

Shelton's theory of separate feeding was based on the research of the famous Russian Scientist Academician Pavlov. These questions interested the doctors of ancient Greece and Egypt. A thousand years ago, Avicenna wrote in his Canon of Medicine, that eating various foods can be harmful, and cause increased weight gain because of the simultaneous digestion of each of them.

However, this theory of separate nutrition became most popular in the early twentieth century, when in 1928, Shelton established a school of health in Texas. There, he began to teach and administer the principles of separate feeding. Over time, the theory began to lose credibility as it was discovered that Shelton did not conduct any scientific study to support his theory.

All he did was to constantly refer to the experience of Academician Pavlov, as the basis of his theory. Academician Pavlov was popular for his discovery of the fact that for each type of food in a dog's stomach, a different composition of digestive juice was allocated.

And this single finding was what served as the source point of Shelton's theory- separate feeding.

Now I feel like I'm boring you with too many details. Well, I am sorry I have to take you through all of this. I consider it important for you to know the rudiments and build-up of this theory, because it is pertinent to the very essence, and the core content of this book.

So, the concept of separate feeding, as theorized by Herbert M. Shelton, is based on the need to separate products into three main groups: proteins, fats and carbohydrates while considering which and what to eat.

According to the author of the system, certain enzymes are necessary for the digestion of a particular product group. For example, an acidic environment is necessary for protein breakdown, and alkaline for carbohydrates. So, what this theory suggests is that, if you do not take this into account, and then you eat two meals from different groups at the same time, then some of them will be digested better, and others worse.

So, an apple eaten on an empty stomach will digest after only 15–20 minutes, but eaten shortly after a meat dish, it will linger in the stomach for longer and begin to ferment, interfering with protein digestion. As a result, both products will enter the intestines poorly processed, which will lead to additional stress on the pancreas and disruption of metabolic processes.

If you eat foods from different groups at different times of the day, all these problems can be avoided. So, according to Shelton, his theory of separate diet can help speed up metabolism, reduce weight and improve the gastrointestinal tract.

However, this theory has been criticized by many, and is believed to be true by others.

But then, like I earlier stated, my theory of separate feeding is quite different from that of Shelton's. I did not use his method of separate feeding to the full extent, as Shelton suggests. But regardless, I can assure you that you will get value for your time spent reading, and money expended in buying the book. Since the aim is to lose weight, let's just pay attention to achieving this with my tested and effective method.

This book will be discussing a process of weight correction mostly dependent on nutrition, and it also thrives on visualization. It is based on the results of a very interesting study conducted by scientists at Columbia University, and has helped me, as well as some of my friends.

INTRODUCTION

Getting rid of obesity has been, and still remains an exciting topic of discussion for many people, especially women. Today there is a huge variety of dietary plans and systems targeted towards weight loss. And with these, it is a normal phenomenon for women to get confused, distracted and sometimes even deceived.

People have so easily forgotten that body systems differ across people, so what works for my sister might not necessarily work for me. In their ignorance, they invest so much money and time, and get significantly different results. But here is a program ideal for you.

Did you just mutter the words "How does she know?" Well, this system is universal, and will work for anybody, so long as you stay dedicated to the program.

So! First, I think we should get acquainted. My name is Lydia, and for me the problem of excess weight was very serious. After the birth of my first child, I gained extra pounds. I didn't like it so I tried different diet plans, but did not get anywhere close to the result I wanted. Of course there were results, but they were very insignificant to the point that sometimes, I could not even understand whether it was a result of a diet, or it was just natural fluctuations in weight.

I consulted with a nutritionist, and I learnt better methods. The effect was much better, but unfortunately, I could not follow through with the process. The diet I was given was tedious, and for me, unrealistic. You know, maybe if I lived alone, it would be easier. But when you have a family - in addition to yourself, you have to prepare food for your husband and child, who do not stick to your diet.

Later on, my daughter fell sick with a very serious diagnosis, and we went to the hospital. I was in the hospital with her for almost a year, and then of course, I had no thoughts about any diet. And almost immediately after my first daughter recovered, our second daughter was born, and after the second birth, my figure certainly did not become any better.

In this book, I will tell you about a very simple and effective method that really helped me. I was able to lose 13-20 pounds per month, and I felt great. I did not have to prepare a separate meal for my husband and children; I did not have to portion my out food daily. I ate the same as usual, but only a little differently.

This method was tested in my own experience and those of some of my friends who also experienced it. Below is a diagram illustrating the major highlights we'll be discussing in the book.

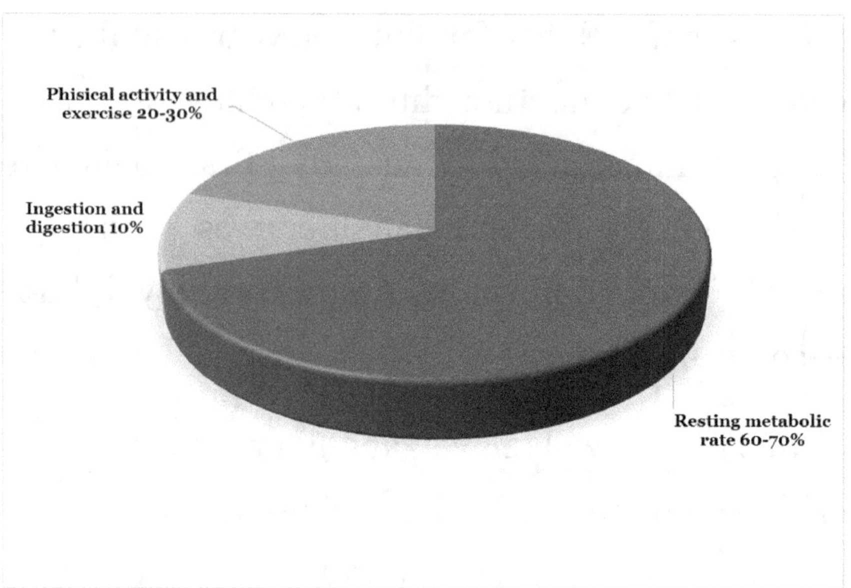

In this diagram, we see the average basic energy consumption of the human body. It explains that most of the total energy is expended on the internal work of the body (resting metabolic rate): the functioning of the internal organs, the work of the brain, the cardiovascular system, and so on.

This means even if you just lie on the couch all the time without even moving your finger, you can still lose weight. As we see, even physical activity affects energy consumption much less. Of course, this does not mean you can give up the gym and physical activity altogether/

In my opinion this is an important point. This 20-30% is also important. I just want to say that even if you don't have time to go to the gym, or at least do the exercises at home, you still have every chance to lose weight and become slim!

Your tool kit will contain:

- Nutrition
- Visualization

I do not need to say a lot about nutrition. As you would have presumed, it is the major tool here, and the book will be dwelling on it a whole lot. As for the visualization, you can certainly do without it, but believe me - it will greatly improve and speed up the process.

It seems to me that today there are not many people who are still not familiar with visualization. And if you still do not know what it is there is a lot of information on this topic on the Internet. Visualization will take you only 2 to 5 minutes at least 2 times a day.

Just sit back and relax, every necessary detail will be explained in the book.

CHAPTER ONE

THE BASIC

Excess weight is a burden for anyone. It increases the stress on the joints, causes difficulty in the functioning of internal organs, puts more stress on the cardiovascular system, and stresses the body in lots of other ways.

So, I would always say weight loss is not just a program to help you lose weight, it is primarily the improvement of our overall health. For some people, the goal of weight loss is basically for beauty and aesthetics, to increase their chances with guys, or improve their self-esteem. But for me, it is first a call to sound health before all of those.

This chapter will be discussing the concepts basic to this study. And to start with, it will briefly discuss the two major tools with which we will be fighting obesity.

Nutrition

We all know very well we cannot do without food. It is through food where we get the vital nutrients our body needs, and operates with. We need vitamins, minerals, proteins, fats, and carbohydrates, and in the event these nutrients are stored up wrongly, (for instance fats being stored in the stomach) then it will be safe to say there is an indication of trouble. So, while we will be talking about weight loss, we should understand that being overweight is not the only problem of malnutrition.

If you follow the advice in this book, you will certainly lose weight. In my case, I lost 13-20 pounds per month, and sometimes even more. But later in my weight loss journey, I realized losing weight was just a bonus and a consequence of a general improvement in the condition of my body.

It may seem to you that 13 pounds per month is not so much, but I want to immediately warn you that extremely fast weight loss often causes damage to your health. In addition, after this, people very often start to gain weight again. Our goal is to effectively help you achieve a sustainable weight loss plan and help you reach a weight level you have set for yourself, one whose results you can keep for life.

So, with nutrition, the factors we will be working with are the required proportion of each food nutrient, how it should be eaten, and when it should be eaten. These factors will be used to influence the change in weight desired.

Visualization.

Choose a couple of minutes at a particular time of the day, daily, preferably at a time when you think there is no one else except you at home, or just go to another room. There, get a chair or stool, sit in it, turn off distractions, meditate and get a picture of you in your desired weight size and do the following.

- Prep yourself mentally:

The following is a mental exercise I will advise you to engage in. It is optional though important. Now, here it is:

First, try and create a virtual vacuum cleaner in your head. Create with an incredible performance of let's say 500% or 1000% power. Now give yourself a quick reminder that the vacuum cleaner you created is aimed at improving your whole body's weight, to improve the work of all your internal organs and essentially reduce your weight to your desired size.

Do not gloss over that step. It might sound silly, but I urge you to just do it anyways, there is no harm in trying it out. So, after creating it, imagine that this machine is being used to clear out all the unnecessary elements in your body.

Do this imaginative exercise, and be as clear as possible. Imagine how you take the handle of this vacuum cleaner and begin to hold it over every part of your body, and especially on the most problematic ones. As clearly as you can, imagine putting the vacuum cleaner over a part of your body, and see that this part has gotten smaller and become thin and graceful.

After you have removed all this excess fat from all over your body, imagine that a powerful fire is burning in front of you and you are emptying all of the fat into the fire. Now tell yourself your bag of fat is all burned up in this fire and so now has no chance of returning.

You can visualize with open eyes or you can close your eyes, whatever you prefer. Personally, I was comfortable doing it with my eyes closed. By the way, I will share with you a little trick, which will be especially useful for women. If you do not want absolutely all parts of your body to shrink, for example, you do not want to lose weight in your breasts, then in your imagination, you can picture not vacuuming your breasts! In some cases, you can always imagine turning on the reverse button and put back a bit of what the vacuum cleaner pulled out of you! Chest or butt, wherever you want.

The above procedure should be carried out at least twice a day, and preferably more often.

And the second phase of visualization you need to do, will be done before each meal, and it will take you just a few seconds. Before any meal, even if it is just an apple, mentally tell yourself:

"Thank God or the universe (which option is closer to you) for the food you sent me. I ask you to share the energy I will get from this food with all the needy and the hungry"

I repeat once again that you don't have to do the visualization, but I assure you that it works awesomely well!

CHAPTER TWO

NUTRITION

Now that we are getting into the main bone of contention, I'll need you to settle down and concentrate. In this chapter, we will be discussing the pattern in which nutrition is supposed to follow, for it to affect the kind of change we desire in the body. So let me remind you that this book is on separate feeding, but as I already stated, it is not a total offshoot of the principle of separate feeding, so sit back while I explain all about this principle I am about to discuss with you.

Let me start by asking you how heavy your usual meals always are daily, and how often you eat these meals?

Well, with weight loss as the goal in mind, you can decide to follow either of these plans.

You eat in very little portions, but often. Like as frequently as five times in a day.

Eat one or two heavy meals daily, and on some days, fast.

Both plans will get you to lose weight, only at different speeds. The first option, for instance, will get you to lose weight faster, and more drastically when compared to consuming heavy meals in the second option. So always bear in mind that sometimes, it is not always about the quantity of food, but about the methodology of eating.

With close scrutiny of both options I have shown above, I guess by now you must be wondering about their differences. This is because; eating light five times, and eating large once, should still amount to the same quantity, yea? Well, this is to show that weight gain or loss has more to do with the digestion process than it has with your consumption quantity.

But one thing that should be noted is regardless of the fact the first option is the better one, it is not suitable for everyone. This is true because the plan is not flexible. Imagine running the plan on a very busy schedule, one that doesn't give room for much rest time, let alone give you enough time to prepare and eat five times a day. So, sticking to this plan is not for everyone.

But that notwithstanding, this second option will suffice. Remember that the goal of this separate diet program is to help you lose weight without necessarily changing your schedule and lifestyle. So, you don't have to struggle with changing your schedule to fit the plan, rather, the plan will be adjusted to suit you. So, if what you can do is eat only twice a day in large portions, then stick with it, you will still lose weight.

Another important point to note with this plan is your drinking habits. Let's start by analyzing how and when you drink water.

First, make it a habit to always drink a glass of water twenty minutes before a meal. This will help start the digestive process. Yes, the process certainly will not start with a glass of water, but this way, your stomach will already be prepared for eating, and your enzymes will be prepared to get to work.

But this is not a universal rule. If you are eating something really light, like some fruit, or a snack, then it won't be necessary to drink water. Another thing is that it is not good for you to drink water during meals. And not just water, but also any liquid, be it juice, soda, tea, and so on. Asides the fact it takes up space for food, any liquid that enters a stomach with food in it dilutes the gastric acid, and reduces its concentration. And this complicates the digestive process, and stretches the time for digestion of the food.

In some cases, the digestion process even lingers until the time of the next meal. And what this does is that the previous meal will not have time to digest before the next meal. And in the final analysis, the implication of this to the body is unhealthy fat. So, try to abstain from water while eating. And even after eating, don't drink water immediately. Drink water 30 minutes after eating.

So, this is a quick recap:

Drink water 20 minutes before meals (conditional).

Do not drink during the meal.

Drink water 30 minutes after a meal.

Basic Product Compatibility Tips

Now, having talked about your water intake, let's get into the business of the day. Below I will give you the basic principles of the separate food program. For me, it has already become a habit and it is not even comfortable for me to start eating differently now.

So, getting down to the basics, food products are divided into 3 categories. Well, this is according to the principle of separate foods, and they are: proteins, fats, and carbohydrates. But on a quick note, it's important you understand that this statement is not absolutely true, because there is no particular food product that contains just one food nutrient.

Food components will almost certainly contain combinations of protein and carbohydrate; carbohydrate and fats; or fats and protein, although they are usually dominated by one nutrient. As a result of this, there are rules according to how some types of products can be eaten together, while some cannot even be combined with other food products.

In subsequent paragraphs, we will be discussing safe combination tricks. Ones that will aid you in your goal. So below are food classes you should pay attention to, and embrace, if you can.

1. Cereals

Cereals and porridge generally go well with meat, seafood, and even vegetables, so there, we have a viable combination. Cereals and porridge are meals you really should eat. They are a perfect breakfast option, and what's more? They come in several varieties. Especially porridge, it is filling, and is not loaded with calories. It is usually made with a cereal, typically oats. Easy, and fast to prepare on a busy morning.

Porridge for most cultures is traditional, especially in North European Countries. In some countries, instead of oats, barley or other grains are used. It can also be made from corn, or even a mixture of corn flour and sorghum. It can also be made from potatoes, wheat, rice, buckwheat, quinoa, millet, farro, sorghum, rye and spelt, and an endless list of others. It is a meal that is flexible, depending on your preferences.

A bowl of 100g oatmeal porridge, cooked with water will give you about 71kcal. And this remains the same for all types of oatmeal. It is high in whole-grain fiber and protein. It is sugar-free, in as much as you stay away from the flavored ones.

Also, consider rice. It is a very common food in many countries of the world. Many different dishes are made of it and it is usually combined with different things. For instance, Japanese sushi is rice with fish or shrimps, seaweed, and vegetables. And it is a good combination. In the Caucasus, one of the most traditional dishes is called pilaf. It is rice with slices of meat and finely chopped vegetables. And it is also a very good combination.

2. Potatoes

Potatoes are well combined only with other vegetables. In my family, it used to be a common meal item for dinner. We would eat potatoes, a piece of meat, and vegetable salad for dinner. We got used to it so that it became very unusual for us to stop this combination. But now, we eat meat with salad fine, and add more rice or some porridge to it.

By the way, it is wrong to eat cucumbers and tomatoes together, at the same time. Please instead of combining these vegetables, you should just take them separately. But note that generally, cucumbers can be combined with other vegetables, asides tomatoes, and tomatoes can be combined with other vegetables alike, the only itch is putting them together in one salad or in any meal at all.

When I started out on this plan, it was a nightmare for my husband. This is because his favorite salad is cucumbers with tomatoes and olive oil. But he still sadly stayed with the plan. He had to, because I cooked food all at once for the whole family, so George ate with me the way I needed to, on a diet. And of course, I really appreciated his support and thanked him for it, he even lost more than 5 kilograms at some point.

3. Legumes

Beans, chickpeas, soybeans, peas, and other legumes are foods high in vegetable protein, and complex carbohydrates. Legumes are generally a good product for weight loss. They have a fairly low calorie count, which allows you to stay filled and not hungry for a long time after a meal.

But despite the fact that they have low calorie load, they are very nourishing. So, while you are trying to slim down, it is advisable that you do more legume meals. They will provide necessary nutrients needed by the body and at the same time, help you cut down on your calorie load.

But do not over-eat the beans. Excessive consumption of beans may increase the formation of gas in the intestines. Your legume intake should constitute only about ten percent to fifteen percent of the total daily diet daily.

Beans are a leguminous meal with several health benefits. When consumed in the right quantity and often enough, it helps reduce cholesterol in the body, and also decreases blood sugar levels. Beans are a great source of fiber and protein.

There are several variations of beans. Kidney beans is one very healthy type of beans. Like most others, it can be eaten with rice and pretty much any other starchy food. Nine oz of cooked kidney beans will give off 215 Cal.

For combination options, legumes can be combined with any kind of vegetables, except potatoes. This is because starch and protein are not digestion buddies. During the digestion process, starch prevents the absorption of protein. And this is the same reason it is wrong to combine potatoes and meat, or fish or eggs together.

This holds true because all these listed foods are also protein-rich foods, but can be combined with non-acidic fruits and vegetable oil. But take note of the fact you can't combine fish and meat with legumes. It is always easy to miss that, so let me repeat it; legumes should not be combined with meat, fish, or eggs. All three products are rich in protein, so it's better to choose just one food.

4. Fruits

Fruits are full of every good thing. And some of them can be instrumental to weight loss. Bananas for example have 422 milligrams of potassium, and potassium helps to reduce the quantity of sodium in the body, and this eventually reduces belly fat. But the only thing with fruit is timing. They cannot just be eaten any time you want. Fruits should be taken about an hour after a meal. Do not attempt to eat your fruits on an empty stomach or even immediately after eating.

Watch out for fruits. Not all variations of fruits can be combined with other meals or even other foods, and eaten together.

You can try apples and peanut butter. The combination is good for weight loss and is safe. Peanut butter for instance will keep you full with its monounsaturated fat. And apples, which are fiber laden, help to reduce visceral fat. The

Combined with cinnamon toppings is the way to go!

5. Dairy Products and Melon

This duo shouldn't be combined with anything. Now I'm treating them as individual meals and not as a compound food. So, if you drank milk, then the next meal should be no sooner than after 3 hours. The same goes for melons. Although at the expense of dairy products, you could have either hard or soft cheeses.

Now this can be combined with vegetables and with some fruits, like pears, and grapes. Protein sources are very important in your meals. This is because the lack of protein in your diet indirectly leads to fat gain. Yes, it is that important because it helps you stay full, and will keep you away from eating too frequently. Greek yogurt for instance is heavily packed with protein.

Ice cream is a diary product that you will be advised not to take; well, while you are on all those other diets. But with this separate meal diet plan, you get a yes to ice creams! Yea I know, I can relate! So, if you are craving ice cream on a hot day after lunch, then it is fine. Yea, you heard me right. The plan can allow for that.

Remember I told you earlier that while on the plan, you won't have to change your lifestyle as such. In fact, that is what amazes me the most about the diet plan, and what prompted me to share it. I see lots of women get frustrated in their diet plans and just give it all up halfway. Trust me, with how stringent some plans are, it is not impossible to want to quit.

So enough about digressing, what I was going to say is that if you want ice creams so badly, then you can have it. Only that it shouldn't be too often, and for the sake of your figure, and your health, wait at least one hour after meal before taking it.

6. Eggs.

Eggs are a very interesting food product. They contain a lot of protein and lecithin. Protein experts usually refer to eggs as the "ideal protein." And this is due to the fact they contain amino acids in optimal proportions for our body. This is generally one of the best products for breakfast. And those who do not eat eggs for fear of cholesterol, might need to hear this:

- In 2015, scientists in Sweden conducted a large-scale experiment involving about 30,000 people and found out that 1 egg per day does not affect the increase in cholesterol in the body.
- Cholesterol is of two kinds: good (hard) and bad (soft).
- 80% of the cholesterol in our body is produced inside the body, from the numerous processes within the body, while only 20% is gotten from the food we eat.

In general, cholesterol is a rather extensive topic, I cannot afford to discuss it here, but just look out for the book: "7 pillars of optimal health." In this book, I'll give a detailed breakdown of cholesterol. So away from talks about cholesterol, if your health is normal, and there are no special recommendations from a doctor, you can safely eat 6 to 10 eggs a week and it's best of all for breakfast.

While on this diet plan, eating an egg is not a biggie, but remember that eggs can be combined with any vegetable, except potatoes actually. Cooking an egg or omelet for breakfast, especially with tomatoes or broccoli, is a great thing to try. In fact, your stomach and your body will be very grateful to you. Note that fried eggs with bacon are not the best combination, but acceptable. If you really like bacon and eggs, you can have it.

7. Bakery Products

Bakery products are amazing, especially when fresh and warm, but then, they might not be good for you.

Let's imagine you are walking by a street, and then you walk past a bakery. Of course, while passing, you will notice the aroma of the freshly baked bread. What do you do at this point? Because the aroma is always tempting, and you will just feel like buying it and eating it all yea? Especially while it is still warm.

But let me warn you that if you have decided to go on a weight loss journey, then eating fresh bread is not good for you. In fact, it should not be found with you, it is totally wrong to take it. But the good thing is if you are not ready to give up on your love for bread just yet, then here's a tip for you! Get your bread, put it in the fridge for at least 3 days. And after that, you now can safely eat it.

For you to revive the taste, you can heat it up in a toaster. The explanation for this is fact is that the yeast fungi which is in fresh bread is an active contributor to the deposition of fat in the body, especially fat on the sides. But once the bread has been left in the refrigerator for 3 days, the number of yeast fungi in the bread will have reduced to a bearable minimum and so you can enjoy hot toast without the risk of gaining weight.

8. Butter

During this period when we are working towards weight loss, it is better to refuse butter. So that your weight-loss program doesn't get upset. So, when you reach your weight goal, then you can resume consumption of butter.

Have you noticed the looks of regular customers of fast food restaurants? You have not? I think you really should start observing! They mostly don't eat healthy. You can often see them order a burger, then fries, and drink it all down with a sweet soda. Now, from the point of view of proper nutrition, there is no iota of healthy eating habits being displayed. The combinations are not right; the nutritional load of the food is not healthy. In fact, everything is wrong with the food.

When you have potatoes, meat, fresh bread, almost no vegetables and a lot of sugar, all on one plate, and you still want to take ice cream or milk shake for dessert. such eating habits are wrong.

9. Pasta

Pastas are a delicious lot. There are several variants of pastas, but common among these variants are- Spaghetti, Tortellini, Ravioli, Penne, Fettuccine, Orzo, and Macaroni. These pastas can be made into different meals, and best of all, they can be combined with fish, seafood, and vegetables. Pastas can be whole grained or refined. So, depending on the choice of the buyer, both variations are always available in the market. But like I said earlier, while on the separate meal diet plan, it is advisable for you stick to whole grain pastas.

Whole-grain pasta is renowned for its fiber, manganese, selenium, copper, and phosphorus contents, and it will help curtail your cravings and appetite. In order to get the best out of a pasta meal, you could combine it with protein sources of your choice, but avoid combining it with meat. And note that you have to be careful when choosing toppings for your pasta. Choose toppings low in fat contents. You could have heart-healthy vegetables too. But remember that when it comes to pasta, moderation is key.

Pasta is a high carb meal and therefore shouldn't be taken in large quantities or too often. So, while taking in only occasionally, make sure to take it with healthy toppings.

In general, these types of products are well combined with each other, and they can be combined in different ways. Now because they are usually well combined, the products are perfectly digested together and would not interfere with one another. So, this suggests that not all foods can be combined without having issues.

All of the above are basic product compatibility tips, according to my separate feeding program. So, if you wish, you can of course use these tips, or follow the principle of separate feeding more carefully, and stick to the rules. But you should understand that the ideal principles of separate feeding, unlike those of mine, will bring additional discomfort to your usual life. Those recommendations listed above are quite enough. If you stay with it, you will definitely get results. Remember, I discovered its potency from my own experience, and from those of my friends.

So, conclusively, let me re-mention, and in the process, remind you briefly, about what your action plan should look like, on this journey towards your ideal figure.

- ❖ First visualization several times a day. You remember, yea?
- ❖ Give thanks before every meal.
- ❖ Drink your water rightly, a glass of water 20 minutes before meals.
- ❖ And finally, be careful of your food combinations, eat the right mix of foods.

Do all of these, and you will succeed!

The Extras

In addition to all of the discussed topics, I will want to touch on another discussion. Here, I will discuss the extras that can help you speed up your weight loss journey. So, let's discuss 3 main points.

Water

Not many people know this, but a very common cause of obesity in women is not overweightness, but edema. The body is experiencing a shortage of water and begins to keep it in reserve. Obesity, of course, too, but edema is also quite common. Or the combination of obesity and edema is just in my case, as I had both of these problems at once.

And edema arises not from an excess of water, but from its lack. You have often heard that you need to drink 8 cups of water per day. This is not just a faceless recommendation; it is really very important! The body must receive enough water to flush out toxins. So, the optimal dose of water for you can be calculated by a simple formula: 0.5 ounces of water multiplied by the number of your pounds.

It is clear that if your weight is 100 kg, then drinking a little more than gallon of water per day is quite difficult. But at least try to drink 8 cups a day. For example, my husband George is my big man. His height is 6.3 feet and his weight is just 220 pounds. He does not drink 12.5 cups of water a day, but he drinks 8 cups, some days more.

By myself I can say that at the beginning it was not easy to drink 8 cups per day. I just could not pour in so much water. And every 15 to 20 minutes I had to run to the toilet. In the first week, or two, I even gained a little weight, because the body, out of habit, continued to store water. But then the body realized there were no problems with water and began to work as expected.

The edema began to slowly go away, and after a couple of weeks I was already used to drinking so much water. I was even uncomfortable if I did not drink water for a long time. A very important point. When we talk about the need to drink water, we mean pure water. Tea, coffee, juice, even if you just add a little lemon to the water - do not fit.

If there is anything other than water in water, then it is a solution for our body. In this form, it cannot use water, so our body first deals with the separation of the solution into the water and everything else. Clean water entering the body is immediately used for its intended purpose- it partly goes to domestic needs, and the rest is used to remove toxins and other debris.

All the excess is dissolved in water, that is, the body makes its solution and brings it out. At the exit, we see this solution, which is called urine. In general, you need to drink at least 8 cups of water per day. To make it easier, upload an application to your Smartphone that will remind you to drink some water.

Sugar

Sugar is generally the worst enemy of the body. Ok, let me rephrase that. Excess sugar is generally one of the worst enemies of the body. It tampers with your figure and can mess with your health. Today, some scientists even call it a drug. I will not elaborate on the subject matter of sugar and its effect on your health, in this book.

If you are interested in reading all about sugar, then you can check out my book "7 pillars of optimal health." The details can be found there. As for the question of losing weight, it is important to know that sugar is a very fast carbohydrate. This means the feeling of hunger is quenched for a very short time.

So having eaten one candy, in a matter of minutes, you will begin to crave another, and would be moved to eat the second, and then the third and so on. An adult can control himself and confine himself to a few candies, but what will a child do if he is left alone with the candies? Of course, he will eat them until they run out.

Plus, the sugar is very high in calories. Today, people eat too much sugar, even without realizing it. It is used almost everywhere in the food industry. Baking, pastry, ketchup, sauces, any canned food, yogurt and so on. There is a huge amount of sugar in sweet soda and oatmeal, which many give to their children for breakfast.

My family and I have very limited sugar intake. There are practically no sweets at home; we drink tea without sugar at all. There was a time when we had to visit one of our friends whom we had not seen for a long time. At their residence, we were offered tea. When George was done pouring the tea, two spoons of sugar was added to his tea, as that was how he always had his tea before now. But that day, my husband could not drink his tea, he had to order another cup of tea without sugar. He was already accustomed to drinking tea without sugar, so much so that sweet tea made him nauseated.

By the way, I will tell you one more life hack. How do you cook a delicious cake? Take any cake recipe, divide the amount of sugar into two and you still get a great cake. Are you in doubt? I'd advise you to try it out first, as you'll only discover that sugar doesn't make a great cake.

In general, if you are a lover of sugary things, then you should seriously think about this issue, and cook up a way around cutting down on your sugar intake. Sugar causes great damage to the figure, and even more harm to health.

- **Sport**

Remember the graph of energy consumption at the beginning of the book? So, the 20% the body spends on physical activity should not be ignored. 20% is a good number, a non-negligible addition to the result. In addition to the extra pounds dropped, it will also increase your tone, speed up your rate of metabolism and improve your overall well-being.

First, your body will start to burn stored glycogen for energy, so there will be a decrease in the stored up fat. And after consistent exercise and sporting, your body will start to burn mainly fat.

While exercising, concentrate on cardio activities, weightlifting and resistance training. The latter ones will help Increase muscle mass, and this will help you burn more calories and raise your basic metabolic rate.

Gymnasium, swimming pool, yoga will also be excellent fitness choices for you. You can even alternate these types of physical activity. Walk a few months to the gym, then a few months to the pool or somewhere else.

Do you know where the fat goes from the body? It does not turn into muscles, as many believe. In fact, in the process of burning fat, the fat is oxidized and then it decomposes into carbon dioxide and water. We exhale carbon dioxide, and water is either excreted in the urine or excreted in the form of sweat.

So, as you know, the gym will help you speed up the process of losing weight. With rapid breathing and sweating, you can be sure these are the signs that fat has begun to burn. But I think I should chip this in- while you are sweating profusely, and breathing heavily, know that your lungs, your heart, and some other organs of the body are being forced to ramp up different functions at the same time, and this could lead to serious consequences during exercise if they are not cooled off with water.

Another thing to note is that water helps muscles, connective tissues, and joints to move correctly. So, the point is for you to always drink water before, during, and after exercise to avoid dehydration. When you stay hydrated during exercises, you kill the risks of falling victim to such things as muscle cramps and fatigue. So, keeping water close at hand is essential, especially if you are exercising in hot, humid, or very sunny conditions.

CHAPTER THREE

HOW DOES IT WORK?

Wow, you made it down here, I must say congratulations, as you have gone through the bulk of the book. But before you go on, I will need you to do me a favor.

I want you to go over all of your jottings, refresh your mind, and see if you are still up to date with what the book is dishing out. If not, I'll advise you go back over whichever part of the book that you have not absorbed, and do a reread.

I guess now that you have done that, we are refreshed enough to continue this journey. So, I'll start this chapter by giving you this interesting narrative, and we'll kick off from there.

Do you know how the body works? Or let me narrow it down. Do you know how the digestive system in the body works? Or better still, I guess I should just spill it as- how you get the feeling of hunger? I bet you don't know.

So, in general, the feeling of hunger is a typical signal of the body. It is nothing serious, it is only a method with which the body communicates a sensation of low amount of food substances in the body. And interestingly enough, this 'sensation' is usually about 'food nutrients', and not 'food'; and this is contrary to what some people would suppose.

The popular narrative is that everybody that is hungry, is hungry because their stomachs are empty. And you'll hear people say, "I get hungry easily these days oh!" But then, that is not the case. The real thing is the majority of us have not sat down, and taken time out to understand the language of their body.

Learn this today, that hunger doesn't necessarily mean lack of food, it just might be the lack of a particular food nutrient.

So let me explain what I mean. Your body understands this, that the only way to get the necessary trace elements for itself is when you eat something. So, when our body is in urgent need of some elements: some specific vitamins, minerals, or even if it's just a need for more protein. Then, the next line of action for the body is to make you feel hungry.

That is the only way it understands. So, for instance, assume you had pizza for lunch, and at that instance when you had pizza, you satisfied your hunger. For a while, while the body digests this pizza, you will feel full. But after a certain period of time, the digestion process will get completed, and then your brain will receive a kind of report on the nutrients that the digestion process could sap off this pizza.

So, the report goes like this:

Protein - 7

Fats - 5

Carbohydrates - 56

Kcal - 300

Vitamin - 1

Mineral - 3

Now, the brain compares this list with the list our body needs to function properly. And it sees that proteins are obtained, fats are obtained, carbohydrates are even in abundance, but there are almost no vitamins, and there are very few minerals, and so on.

The brain realizes that with this meal, the essentials were not completely received. And now, the only option it is left with is to send a new request for food. And there again, guess what we have? Hunger!! There is a feeling of hunger.

But in our ignorance, as a rule, we do not realize what exactly our body is asking us to do. So, we then go all out and load it up with all of the unnecessary nutrients, again leaving the needed ones out. And again, in few hours, we are hungry.

Only in rare cases do people know what to do with their hunger situations. At best, what the body can do is to create cravings. So, after a while, you will see yourself suddenly craving an apple, or an orange. Pay attention to what is your body sending you hints as to what it needs.

The body is a large and very complex mechanism, and for it, each bolt and each gear carry out its role, serving some purpose. Therefore, of course, ideally, it uses a variety of foods to satisfy all the needs of the body.

Food and Body Fat

Body fat is not a terrible thing. I know you'll disagree, but then, it is not. It is the excess of body fat in the body that is a problem. The bottom line is that any food wrongly combined, or eaten in excess, will lead to fat gain. This means that the body requires food nutrients in definite quantities, so if at any point you overeat any of these food nutrients, then you'll begin to add weight. So, whether your diet is high in fat or high in carbohydrates, if you frequently consume more energy than your body uses, you're likely to put on weight.

Below is a succinct account of the relationship that each food nutrient shares with body fat.

Carbohydrate and Body fat

Carbohydrate shares a positive relationship with body fat, so the more your intake of carbohydrate, the more body fat you'll get. In fact, carbohydrate constitutes more body fat than fatty meals do. This is regardless of the fact that carbohydrates, in comparison to fat are low in calories. On average, one gram of carbohydrates contains four calories, while one gram of fat contains nine calories. Of all the kinds of food nutrient, they are the quickest source of energy. They quickly increase the level of blood glucose.

Protein and Body fat

Protein is a body building food. Note that it builds muscles not fat. Another thing it does is to change the level of some weight regulating hormones. So, protein has a strong relationship with body fat.

Another thing I need you to note is that weight loss doesn't necessarily equal fat loss. In most cases, while trying to lose weight, your muscle mass also goes off along with body fat. Meanwhile, what you really want to lose is body fat. Both the subcutaneous fat (under the skin) and the visceral fat (around organs). But usually, losing muscle is a side effect of weight loss. But then it is one that can be controlled. So, this is one of the ways in which protein becomes useful in body fat loss.

Remember that protein builds energy and repairs worn out tissues, so in the event when you are burning body fat, a high intake of protein will help you keep up an effective fat loss plan. And this is how:

I'm sure you must have seen some people who got into a dietary plan, or hit the gym, or even did both, and actually lost body fat, but then are still looking good; lean and fit. Wow, you'll envy those ones.

But then on the other side of the narrative, I've met people who did all of the above mentioned things and then are looking like shadows of themselves, skinny is not just word to describe it.

Well, in this situation, it will be safe to say the amount of protein intake of persons in these two categories will be a major factor in the different look they came up with. So, without the right amount of protein intake, you may end up looking "skinny-fat" instead of fit and lean.

And that's not all. Protein in itself also causes weight loss, although not as fast as the other macro nutrients will, but the good thing with protein is that it cuts down body fats even without the need for calorie counting or carb restriction and it prevents weight regain. So, at this point, you really cannot go wrong with protein. Eat enough and combine it rightly.

Fats & Oils and Body Fat

Against popular beliefs, fat is not like the major culprit of body fat creation. It does not automatically follow that the amount of fat you take in will constitute the amount of body fat in your body. Some pundits even argue that carbohydrate has the tendency to give off more body fat than fat will.

Fat takes longer time to digest when compared to other foods, and just like carbohydrate, the amount of time varies based on the type of fat.

Once fat is broken down during digestion, some of it gets used right away for energy, and the rest is stored. So, whenever the body needs extra energy, it'll break down the stored fat for energy. The evil here now is when the fat keeps getting stored up, and is not used up.

So, what this means is that fatty foods should be taken in moderation, and combined with more of proteineous foods. Remember that combination is key.

Water and Body Fat

Hmm, it is interesting to know that water also contributes to weight loss. But it shouldn't be to you because I already mentioned it in earlier chapters. Different studies have shown to a large extent the positive correlation that exists between increased water consumption and weight loss. And besides the actual process of weight loss, hydration is key for many factors that play a role in weight loss, including digestion and muscle function.

Drinking water helps boost your metabolism, cleanses your body of waste, and acts as an appetite suppressant, and these are the ways in which it can be channeled to help improve weight loss. It can help you take up space in the stomach, thereby leading to a feeling of fullness and reduced hunger.

In a study carried out in 2014, 12 people who drank 500 mL of cold and room temperature water experienced an increase in energy expenditure. They burned between 2 and 3 percent more calories than usual in the 90 minutes after drinking the water. Just make it a habit to drink at least one 8-ounce glass of water with each meal. Another quick one- drinking cold water may further enhance water's calorie-burning benefits, because the body expends energy, or calories, by heating up the water for digestion.

Body Fat and Muscles

I just thought to clarify this, and do it now. Your body does not, and cannot, convert fat to muscle or convert muscle to fat. It is an impossible process and so I'll want you to re-orientate your mind. Simply put, your body can't turn fat into muscle.

You'll find some people saying they are trying to convert their excess body fat into muscle, so they can look fit. Well, this is for you, if you are of that mentality too.

Fat and muscle are composed of two different types of tissue. And it happens that none of both tissue types can be directly converted to the other. It is just like trying to make an orange from a pear.

The only way around this is to first lose fat and then gain weight by building muscle. This will mean that you first start to expend more calories than you take in.

But to lose fat without also losing muscle, you have to eat the right foods: If you cut your calorie intake and don't eat enough protein, weight loss can result in a decrease in not only fat but also muscle.

CONCLUSION

Obesity is an unhealthy phenomenon. If allowed, it can wreck countless havocs within the body. So, before it gets to that point when it becomes really serious and lethal, it is necessary that it is put in check.

Over the years, there have been several methods of combating obesity. While some have proven effective, some others have been recorded to do very little in trying to get rid of excess fat. A lot of people go through so much fussing and stress, all in the name of trying to get rid of excess fat. But then, for some other people, slimming down for them is a call to a totally new life. This is true, as they have to practically take up new habits and change their lifestyles because of the singular need to burn fat. As you can already tell, this is the major reason that birthed this book.

The book is a product of the compassion I bear for people who are caught up in situations like this.

From reading the book, I'm quite sure you can tell that this book sets a specific goal, which is the loss of excess weight. And the method of execution for achieving this goal is what sets the book on a different pedestal from the other ones that you might have read.

For us, you do not have to thoroughly change your eating habits. This is true because that will not, and has not optimally succeeded in producing required results. All you'll need to do is just watch your combinations.

So, after reading my book, and of course making steps to follow through on the plan, I hope you can gladly say for a fact that now, that you are on a feasible weight loss plan, and therefore don't belong to those groups of people who will get stressed out, and probably frustrated from the demands of their plans.

With this separate feeding program that I explained in this book, you should be able to boast of your weight loss progress in no time, and yes! It's not just going to be about your weight loss success, but the fact that you didn't have to thoroughly change some habits that you were used to, or stop eating some foods that were on an A-list for you. The separate feeding scheme allows all of these, and still gives you the result you deserve.

GLOSSARY

- Drink water 20 minutes before meals (conditional).

- Be careful of your food combinations, eat the right mix of foods.

- Do not drink during the meal.

- Eating fresh bread is not good for you, if you want to shed fat off.

- Drink water 30 minutes after a meal.

- Potatoes are well combined only with vegetables

- For quick weight-loss success, eat in very little portions, but often. Like as many as five times in a day

- 80% of the cholesterol in our body is produced inside the body.

- Eat legumcs oftcn. They are generally a good product for weight loss.

- A very common cause of being overweight in women is not obesity, but edema.